Terms and Conditions

LEGAL NOTICE

Table Of Contents

Foreword

Most daily physical activity is looked at as light to moderate in intensity level. There are particular health advantages that may only be achieved with more strenuous physical action, however.

Betterment in cardiovascular fitness is one illustration. Jogging or running supplies greater cardiovascular advantage than walking at a leisurely pace, for example.

In addition, enhanced fitness doesn't simply depend on what physical activity you do, it likewise depends upon how vigorously and for how long you carry on the activity. That's why it's crucial to exercise inside your target heart rate range when doing cardio, for instance, to reach a certain level of intensity level. Get all the info you need here.

Beautiful Body Essentials
Exercise Tips For That Great Body

Chapter 1:

Exercise Basics

Synopsis

Physical activity is specified as movement that demands contraction of your muscles. Any of the actions we do throughout the day that demand movement — housekeeping, gardening, walking, climbing up stairs — are illustrations of physical activity.

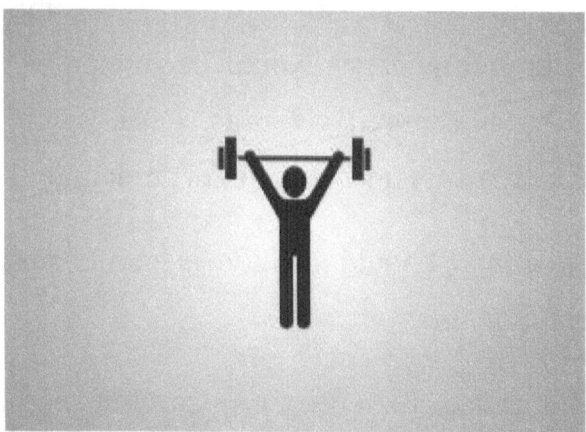

The Basics

Exercise is a particular form of physical activity — planned, purposeful physical activity executed with the intent of gaining fitness or other health advantages. Exercising at a health club, swimming, cycling, running, and sports, like golf and tennis, are all kinds of exercise.

How can you tell if an action is considered moderate or vigorous in intensity level? If you are able to talk although executing it, it's moderate. If you have to stop to catch your breath after saying simply a couple of words, it's vigorous.

Depending upon your fitness level, a game of doubles tennis would likely be moderate in intensity level, although a singles game could be more vigorous. Also, ballroom dance would be moderate, however aerobic dance could be considered vigorous. Once again, it's not simply your choice of activity, its how much effort it demands.

Ideally, an exercise regimen should include elements designed to better each of these components:

Cardio-respiratory endurance. Better your respiratory endurance — your ability to engage in aerobics — through actions like brisk walking, jogging, running, cycling, swimming, jumping rope, rowing, or cross-country skiing. As you reach distance or intensity level goals, reset them higher or shift to a different action to keep challenging yourself.

Muscular force. You are able to better muscular strength most efficiently by lifting weights, utilizing either free weights like barbells and dumbbells or lifting machines.

Muscular endurance. Better your endurance with calisthenics (conditioning exercises), weight training, and actions like running or swimming.

Flexibleness. Work to better your level of flexibility through stretching exercises that are done as part of your exercise or through a discipline like yoga or pilates that contains stretching.

Although it's possible to handle all of these fitness factors with a physically active life-style, an exercise program should help you accomplish even greater advantages.

Increasing the sum of physical activity in your daily life is a great beginning — like parking a couple of blocks from your destination to get in a little walking. However to truly accomplish fitness goals, you'll need to incorporate structured, vigorous actions into your schedule to help you accomplish even more of your fitness and health goals.

Chapter 2:

Set Your Goal And Stick To It

Synopsis

Starting or getting back to a workout routine involves more than simply scheduling your exercises and joining a gym. As a matter of fact, it's totally possible to join a gym and never really go, even as those monthly payments appear on your bank statement. I understand this because I've done that a couple of times in my life. Sticking to your goals demands a couple of mental tricks to help keep you going, centered and motivated.

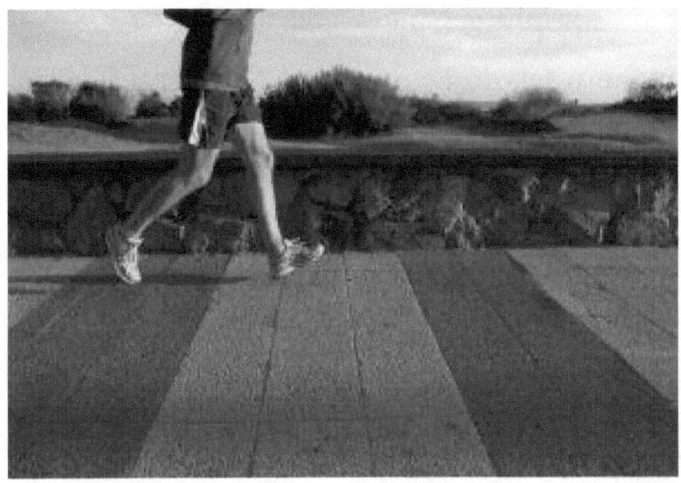

Keep Going

Momentum is a central part of uniform exercise. It's normal to have those weeks when everything goes correctly: You do all your exercises, eat like a health nut and begin to think, 'I may completely accomplish this!'

Then 'it' materializes. 'It' may be a vacation, an illness...something that throws you off your game. Getting back is constantly tough, partly as you've lost that momentum. We already realize that an object at rest tends to remain at rest, so getting going again is the only way to get your momentum moving.

Rather than caring about making up for lost time with intense exercises, center on simply getting some exercise time in. Plan your exercises for the week and call yourself successful simply for turning up.

Purchase yourself a little something like a new pair of running shoes or an exceptional pair of shorts to wear to the gym. If you're having hassles getting back to it, get a new outfit or download a few new songs to your MP3 player so you've something to look forward to.

Make an appointment to exercise with an acquaintance or call your gym and arrange a free consultation with a personal trainer. Even

if you don't sign on, getting back into the exercise environment may be just what you need.

If the thought of coming back to boring gym exercises makes you want to die, do something completely different. Sign on for a local belly dance class or check into that new yoga studio. A switch of scenery and a brand new activity may refresh and rejuvenate you.

Picture this: you're at a party and you've promised yourself you won't scarf down the buffet like a famished maniac. Then you see a huge platter of the prettiest cheese you've ever came across. Many hours later, feeling your cheese hangover start, you vow to make up for it tomorrow with a long workout.

There are some issues with this approach--first, you can't undo what you consumed the night before and, secondly, killing yourself with an exercise isn't a good answer as it makes you hate exercise even more.

If you're busy living in yesterday's errors, many of your decisions will be founded on guilt and shame instead of what you really want (and need) to accomplish to achieve your goals. Real change comes from day-to-day choices and becoming mindful and basing your choices on what you need now (rather than what you did or didn't do yesterday) will make your exercise life much more passable.

Chapter 3:

Get Your Exercise Plan Together

Synopsis

Taking the time to really sit down and make a concrete schedule is the essential first step towards building the body you want. Following comes the tough task of following it each week, but that's a different topic for a different day, for now let's just center on putting a workout schedule together.

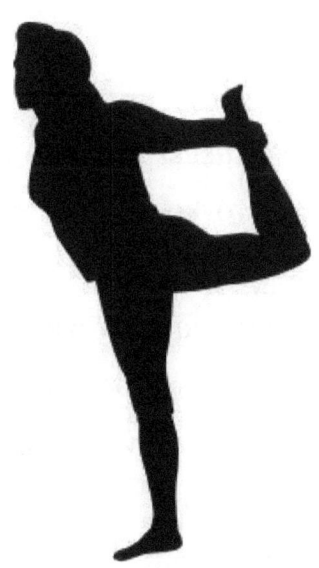

Putting A Plan Together

- Sit with a weekly calendar and ascertain how many days of the week you're willing to workout.
- Choose what particular sort of workout you wish to engage in. For example, cardiovascular workout will help you lose fat, whereas lifting weights will form muscle.
- Devote yourself to exercising according to your plan. This is the most crucial step.
- Abide by your schedule for at the least one month. The gains you'll see after 4 weeks ought to be decent to keep you motivated.

Cardiovascular workout

- Integrate 30-minute workout sessions into your schedule. 30 minutes of every day workouts is enough for most individuals.
- Decide on a sort of cardiovascular workout for a particular day of the week. Utilizing a treadmill or stair-climbing machine, jogging, bicycling, and swimming are all efficient forms of cardiovascular workout.
- Warm up and actively stretch out for five minutes prior to starting any activity.
- Workout at a moderate pace for twenty minutes.
- Follow up with a five minute cool down.

- Switch your schedule to fit longer workout periods if suitable.
- Stick with your schedule.

Weights
- Allow thirty to sixty minute workout sessions for weights. If you don't spend much time socializing or resting during your workout you are able to get a great session of lifting done in that time. Do not rest more than sixty seconds between sets.
- Start by doing total body workouts aimed at conditioning each major muscle group (upper body, lower body and back). Equilibrated development is exceedingly crucial.
- Divide your workouts as you get to be a more experienced lifter. This will enable you to better center on particular muscle groups and areas. A basic split that targets each major muscle group is: chest and triceps, back and biceps, shoulder and legs.
- Rest your muscles in between sessions. Allow each muscle group to rest at least one day between sessions. Your muscles can not grow unless they have time to rest and mend.
- Tailor your agenda to best fulfill your goals.
- Stick with your workout schedule.

Chapter 4:

Make Sure To Warm Up

Synopsis

Many athletes perform some sort of regular warm-up and cool off during training and racing. A suitable warm up may step-up the blood flow to the working muscle which results in diminished muscle stiffness, less risk of trauma and bettered performance. Additional advantages of warming up include physiologic and psychological preparation.

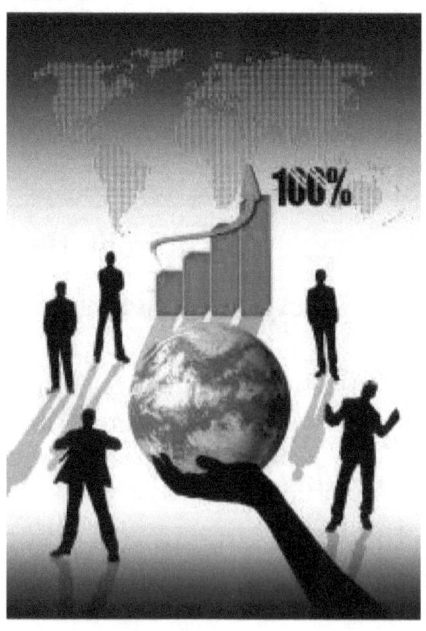

Warm Up

Advantages of a Suitable Warm Up:

Modified Muscle Temperature - The temperature step-ups inside muscles that are utilized during a warm-up routine. A warmed up muscle both contracts more forcefully and loosens up more promptly. In that way both speed and strength may be heightened. Likewise, the chance of pulling a muscle and causing trauma is far less.

Modified Body Temperature - This betters muscle elasticity, likewise cutting back the risk of strains and pulls.

Blood Vessels Enlarge - This brings down the resistance to blood flow and lower strain on the heart.

Better Efficient Cooling - By triggering the heat-dissipation mechanisms in the body (effective sweating) an athlete may cool expeditiously and help preclude overheating early in the event or race.

Modified Blood Temperature - The temperature of blood increases as it goes through the muscles. As blood temperature climbs, the binding of oxygen to hemoglobin de-escalates so oxygen is more readily useable for working muscles, which might better endurance.

Bettered Range of Motion - The range of motion around a joint is modified.

Hormonal Shifts - Your body step-ups its production of assorted hormones responsible for regulating energy production. During warm-up this equilibrium of hormones makes more carbs and fatty acids available for energy manufacturing.

Mental Prep - The warm-up is likewise a great time to mentally prepare for an event by clearing the mind, increasing centering, critiquing skills and technique. Favorable imagery may likewise relax the athlete and establish concentration.

Typical Warm up exercises include:

Bit by bit increasing the intensity of your particular sport. This utilizes the particular skills of a sport and is occasionally called a related warm-up. For runners, the idea is to jog for a while and add a few sprints into the routine to engage all the muscle fibers.

Adding motions not related to your sport in a slow steadfast fashion: calisthenics or flexibility exercises for instance. Ball players frequently utilize unrelated workout for their warm up.

Which to pick? The best time to stretch a muscle is after it has a modified blood flow and has modified temperature to prevent trauma. Stretching out a cold muscle may increase the risk of trauma from pulls and tears.

So you're better off doing gradual aerobic workout prior to stretching. Bear in mind that the best time to stretch is after your workout as your muscles are warm and pliable with the increase of blood in

them. Make certain your warm up starts out gradually, and utilizes the muscles that will be strained during workout.

Keep in mind that the perfect warm up is a very individual process that may only come with practice, experimentation and experience. Try warming up in various ways, at various intensities until you find what works best for you.

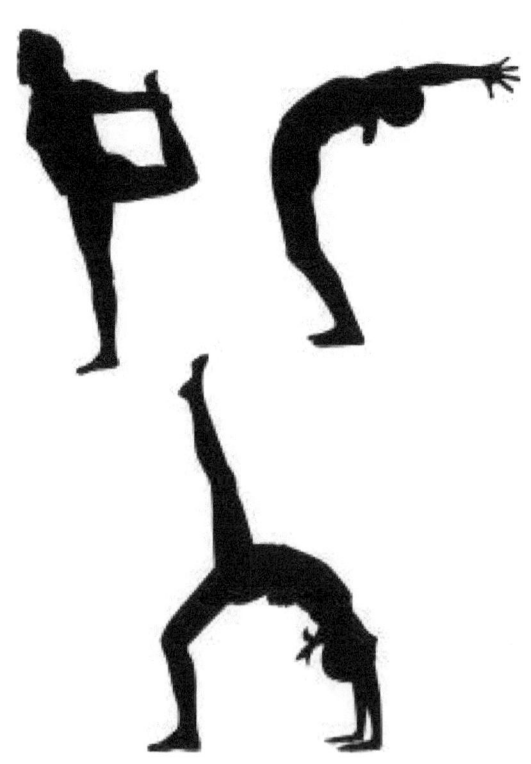

Chapter 5:

Incorporate Cardio Training

Synopsis

With a big share of Americans overweight, it's clear that a lot of us are not abiding by the most recent exercise guidelines dictating up to an hour of exercise every day. In fact, there is no doubt a collective groan when individuals recognized they'd now have to find an hour every day to accomplish something they can't seem to find five minutes for. How crucial are these guidelines and what may you do to make them fit into your life?

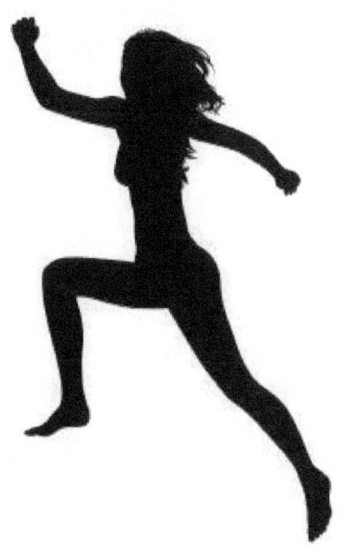

Cardio Basics

Before we get started, you ought to at least know why it's so crucial. Cardiovascular exercise merely means that you're involved in an activity that elevates your heart rate to a level where you're working, but may still talk (also known as, in your Target Heart Rate). Here's why cardio is so crucial:

- It's one way to burn off calories and help you slim down

- It makes your heart strong so that it doesn't have to work as grueling to pump blood

- It step-ups your lung capacity

- It helps bring down risk of heart attack, elevated cholesterol, hypertension and diabetes

- It makes you feel great

- It aids you in sleeping better

- It helps bring down tension

- I could go on all day, however you get the point

Bottom line: you require cardio if you want to get your weight in check and get your tension to a tolerable level.

The opening move is to what kind of activities you'd like to do. The trick is to consider what's accessible to you, what fits your personality and what you'd feel comfy fitting into your life.

If you like to go outside, running, bicycling, hiking or walking are all great choices. If you love the gym, you'll have access to stationary bicycles, elliptical trainers, treadmills, row machines, stair masters and more.

For the home exerciser, there are a number of first-class workout videos to try and you don't require much equipment to get an exceptional home cardio workout.

Bear in mind, you might not know what sort of activity you enjoy yet. That's all part of the experience, so don't be frightened to try something and, if it doesn't work, go on to something else.

Just about any activity will work, provided it demands a motion that gets your heart rate into your Target Zone. Remember:

There's no 'most proficient' cardio exercise. Anything that you like and that gets your heart rate up fills the bill

It's not what you do, but how hard you work. Any exercise may be challenging if you make it that way

Do something you love. If you detest gym workouts, don't force yourself onto a treadmill. If you love socializing, think about sports, group fitness, exercising with an acquaintance or a walking club.

Pick out something you can see yourself doing at least three days a week.

Be flexible and don't be frightened to branch out once you get well-situated with exercise.

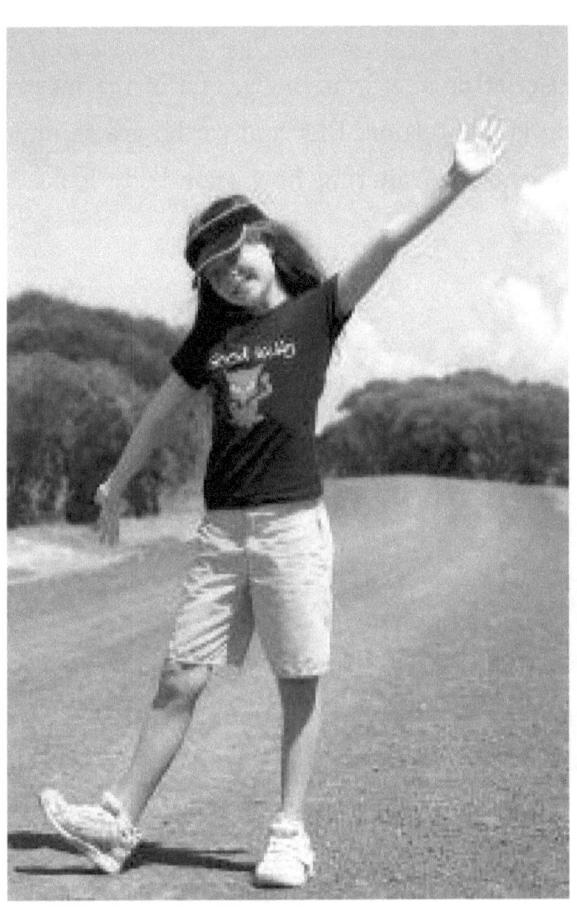

Chapter 6:

Use Weights

Synopsis

If you wish to lose fat or alter your body, one of the most crucial things you can do is lift weights. Diet and cardio are as important, however when it comes to altering how your body looks, weight training wins handily.

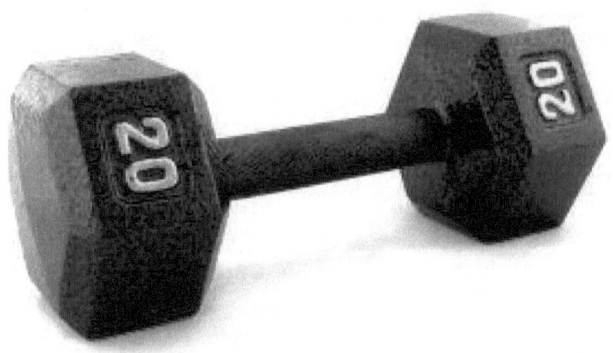

Lifting Basics

If you've hesitated to begin a strength training regimen, it might motivate you to know that lifting weights can:

Help elevate your metabolism. Muscle burns off a lot of calories t, so the more muscle you have, the more calories you'll burn off all day long.

- Fortify bones, particularly crucial for women
- Make you stronger and better muscular endurance
- Help you prevent injuries
- Better your confidence and self-pride
- Better coordination and balance

Getting going with strength training may be confusing--what exercises can you do? How many sets and reps? How much lifting? The routine you pick out will be based on your fitness goals as well as the tools you have available and the time you have for exercises.

If you're establishing your own program, you'll have to understand some basic strength training rules. These rules will teach you how to make certain you're utilizing adequate weight, determine your sets and reps and insure you're always advancing in your workouts.

To build muscle, you have to utilize more resistance than your muscles are used to. This is crucial as the more you do, the more your

body is capable of doing, so you ought to increase your workload to prevent plateaus. In plain language, this implies you ought to be lifting enough weight that you may just complete the desired number of reps. You ought to be able to finish your last rep with difficulty but likewise with great form.

To prevent plateaus (or adaptation), you have to increase your intensity regularly. You are able to do this by increasing the amount of weight lifted, altering your sets/reps, altering the exercises and altering the sort of resistance. You are able to make these alterations on a weekly or monthly basis.

Specificity. This principle means you ought to train for your goal. That means, if you wish to increase your strength, your regimen ought to be designed around that goal (e.g., train with bigger weights closer to your 1 RM (1 rep max)). To slim down, select an assortment of rep ranges to target assorted muscle fibers.

Rest days are even as crucial as workout days. It's during these respites that your muscles grow and change, so make certain you're not working the same muscle groups 2 days in a row.

Before you get going on setting up your routine, keep a couple of key points in mind:

Constantly warm up before you begin lifting weights. This helps get your muscles warm and prevent trauma. You may warm up with light

cardio or by doing a light set of every exercise before moving to heavier weights.

Elevate and lower your weights slowly. Don't utilize momentum to lift the weight. If you have to swing to get the weight up, probabilities are you're utilizing too much weight.

Don't hold your breath and make certain you're utilizing full range of motion throughout the motion.

Stand up straight. Pay attention to your posture and use your abs in every motion you're doing to keep your balance and protect your spine.

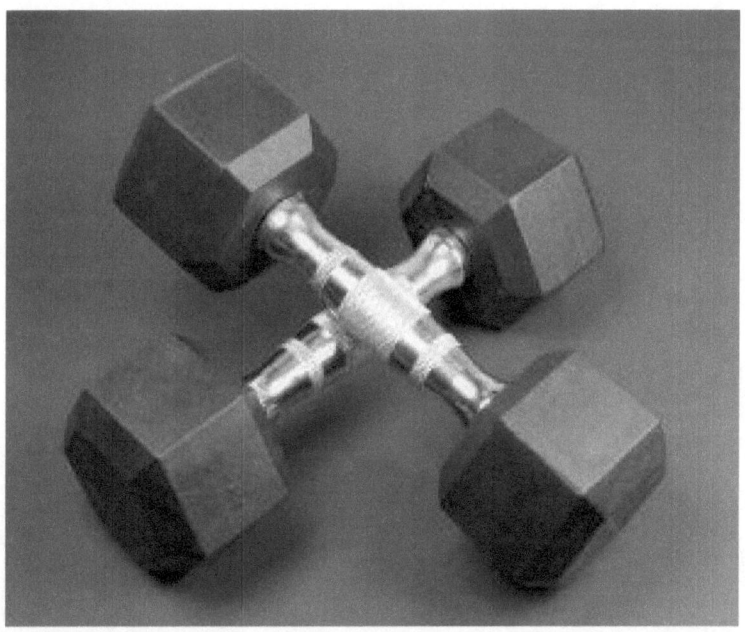

Chapter 7:

Eat Healthy

Synopsis

Healthy eating isn't about rigorous nutrition doctrines, remaining unrealistically thin, or stripping yourself of the foods you like. Instead, it's about feeling good, having more energy, steadying your mood, and keeping yourself as healthy as you can– all of which may be accomplished by learning a few nutrition basics and utilizing them in a way that works for you. You may expand your range of healthy food selections and learn how to plan ahead to produce and maintain a tasty, healthy diet.

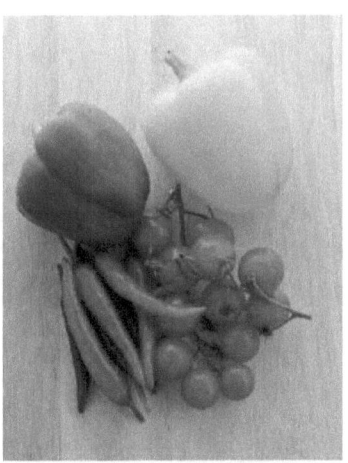

Good Habits

To set yourself up for success, consider planning a healthy diet as a number of little, manageable steps instead of one big drastic shift. If you approach the shifts gradually and with dedication, you'll have a healthy diet sooner than you believe.

Rather than being overly concerned with calculating calories or measuring portion sizes, consider your diet in terms of color, assortment, and freshness.

This way it ought to be easier to make healthy selections. Center on finding foods you love and simple recipes that incorporate a couple of fresh ingredients. Step by step, your diet will get healthier and more delicious.

Begin slow and make shifts to your eating habits over time. Attempting to make your diet sound overnight isn't realistic or bright. Shifting everything at once commonly leads to cheating or quitting on your new eating program.

Make little steps, like adding a salad (full of different color veggies) to your diet once a day or changing from butter to olive oil while cooking. As your little changes become habit, you are able to continue to add sounder choices to your diet.

Each change you make to better your diet matters. You don't have to be perfect and you don't have to totally do away with foods you enjoy to have a sound diet.

The long term goal is to feel great, have more energy, and reduce the risk of cancer and disease. Don't let your stumbles derail you—each healthy food selection you make counts.

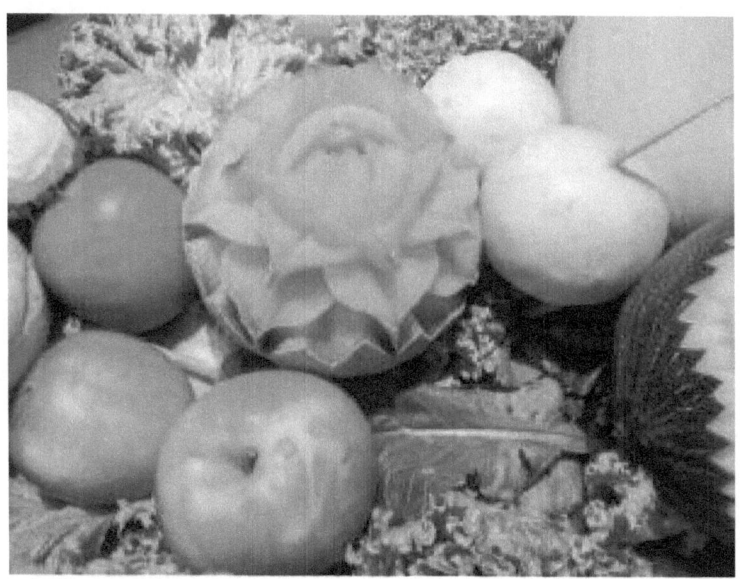

Chapter 8:

The Benefits To A Healthy Lifestyle Other Than Looking Great

Synopsis

The first advantage of living a healthy life-style is that you likely will live a longer and healthier life. If you have a family to support this is really important as you'll be there for them to supply financial and emotional support.

If you have a son or daughter I'm sure that they'll want their mom and dad to be there for them.

For parents you get the joy of raising your youngsters and watching them grow from tot to their early childhood years and all the way up to maturity.

As a parent you'll have the joy of being around your grand kids and even watch them grow.

Advantages

A different advantage of a healthy life-style is that you'll be more vibrant and have more energy. You'll have more get up and go. This will let you be more active and achieve more. This will allow you to have a more favorable attitude in life and will help out your physical, emotional and mental frame of mind.

It will let you be more productive at home and at work. You will not have as many sick days at work therefore making you a more generative employee. If you have a business, this expanded productivity may help your company be more fruitful. Overall this expanded productivity may result in great financial dividends for you in the future.

Overall you'll look and feel better. You'll have a much more positive outlook on life. It will pay dandy dividends for you down the road as far as your physical, emotional and mental frame of mind. It will bring down tension and stress. It likewise will ease and decrease the chances of depressive disorder or getting depressed all the time as you are feeling great about yourself and have a more positive frame of mind.

It's a form of preventive health care and preventative medicine. It will help prevent heart conditions, cancer and many additional debilitating diseases.

I'm saving the best for last. Among the greatest advantages of living a healthy lifestyle is the amount of cash you'll save. When you're healthy you'll;

- Spend less time and cash on physician visits
- Spend less cash on prescriptions
- Fewer if any visits to the hospital
- Lessen the risks of out of control medical expenses which is among the leading causes of bankruptcy and financial destruction.

Regrettably, very few individuals recognize and understand the advantages that a healthy life-style may have on ones bank account.

So these are the advantages of healthy lifestyle and overall how to live a healthy life-style.

Wrapping Up

Bear in mind that there's more to a beautiful body than just utilizing effective wellness products. You need to be on a total preventative healthcare and wellness program that involves diet, nutrition (making a point that your body gets the proper nutrients) and exercise.

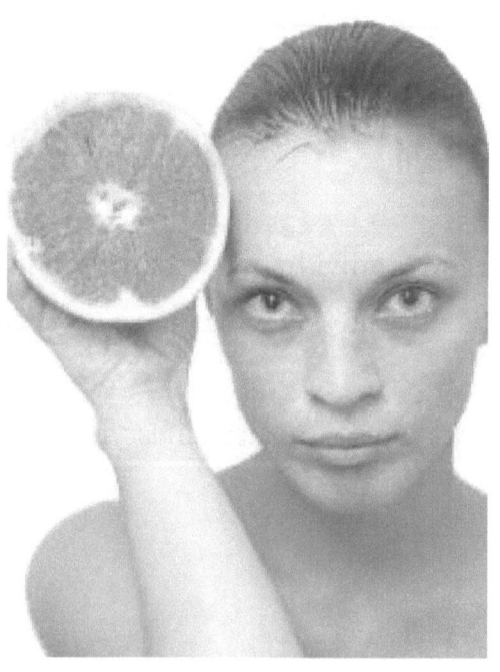

www.ingramcontent.com/pod-product-compliance
Lightning Source LLC
Chambersburg PA
CBHW050525290526
45786CB00007B/2694